The ADHD Solution

Practical Strategies for Kids to Thrive

Raya Curtis

The
ADHD
Solution

Samantha Jameson

Table Of Content

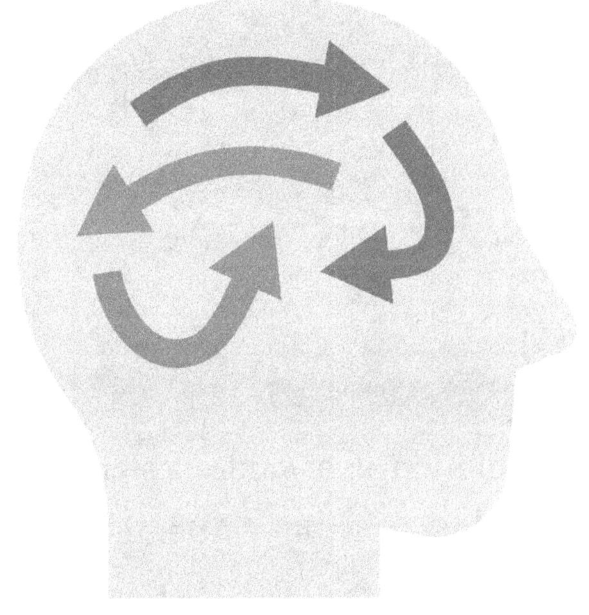

Introduction

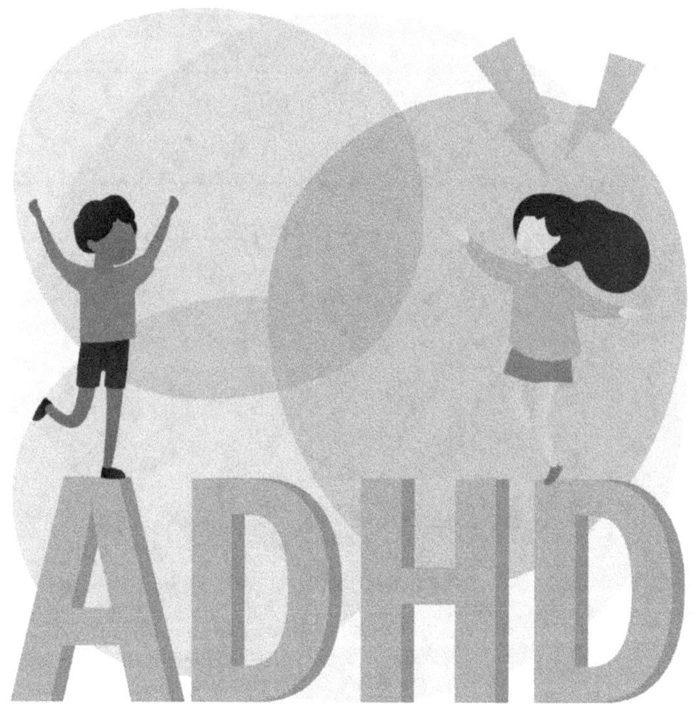

The ADHD Solution is a guide designed to help those struggling with Attention Deficit Hyperactivity Disorder (ADHD) better understand their condition and learn effective strategies to manage their symptoms. The book provides a thorough overview of ADHD, its causes, symptoms, diagnosis, and treatment options, as well as practical advice for making lifestyle changes and finding support.

At the same time, The ADHD Solution is also a celebration of the resilience, creativity, and potential of those living with ADHD. Through stories of both adults and children who have persevered despite the challenges of ADHD, the book provides an inspiring and uplifting vision of what is possible. The ADHD Solution is a valuable resource for anyone looking for information, guidance, and support in managing their ADHD.

ADHD-Friendly Life

Creating an ADHD-friendly life for your child can be a challenging and rewarding task. The goal is to create an environment in which your child can thrive, while also managing their symptoms of

Attention Deficit Hyperactivity Disorder (ADHD). Here are some tips for creating an ADHD-friendly life for your child:

1. Create a routine: Establishing a consistent routine for your child can help provide structure and predictability, which can be beneficial for children with ADHD. This can include a regular bedtime, school and homework times, and time for fun activities.

2. Break down tasks: Large tasks or projects can be overwhelming for children with ADHD, so break them down into smaller, more manageable steps. This can help your child stay focused and on track.

3. Encourage physical activity: Exercise can help children with ADHD to focus and manage their energy levels. Encourage your child to participate

in physical activities that they enjoy, such as team sports, individual sports, or other forms of physical activity.

4. Provide a distraction-free environment: Minimize distractions such as TVs, radios, and other noise-making devices when your child is doing homework or studying. It can also help to create a designated study area that is calm and free from distractions.

5. Limit screen time: Too much screen time can be detrimental for children with ADHD, so it is important to set limits. Encourage your child to spend time doing activities such as reading, playing an instrument, or engaging in creative activities instead.

6. Offer rewards and incentives: Positive reinforcement can be an effective way to help motivate your child to stay focused and on task. Rewards and incentives can be used to encourage good behavior and help your child stay on track.

Creating an ADHD-friendly life for your child may not be easy, but it is possible. With consistency and dedication, you can create an environment in which your child can thrive and reach their full potential.

7. Seek professional help: If needed, seek out professional support from a mental health professional to help your child manage their ADHD. This can help to ensure that your child is getting the best care possible.

8. Talk to your child: Finally, it is important to talk to your child about their ADHD. Let them know that it is okay to struggle and that you are here to support them. This can help them to feel more comfortable and empowered to manage their ADHD.

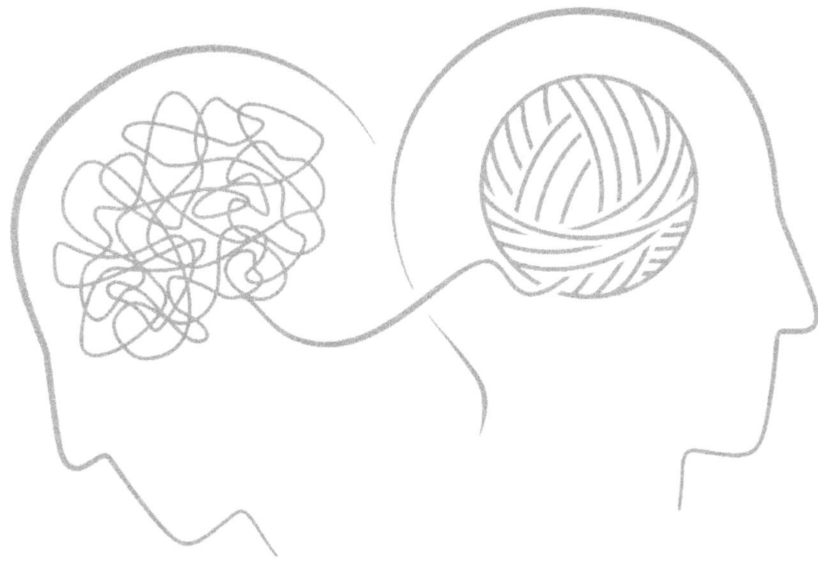

Chapter 1

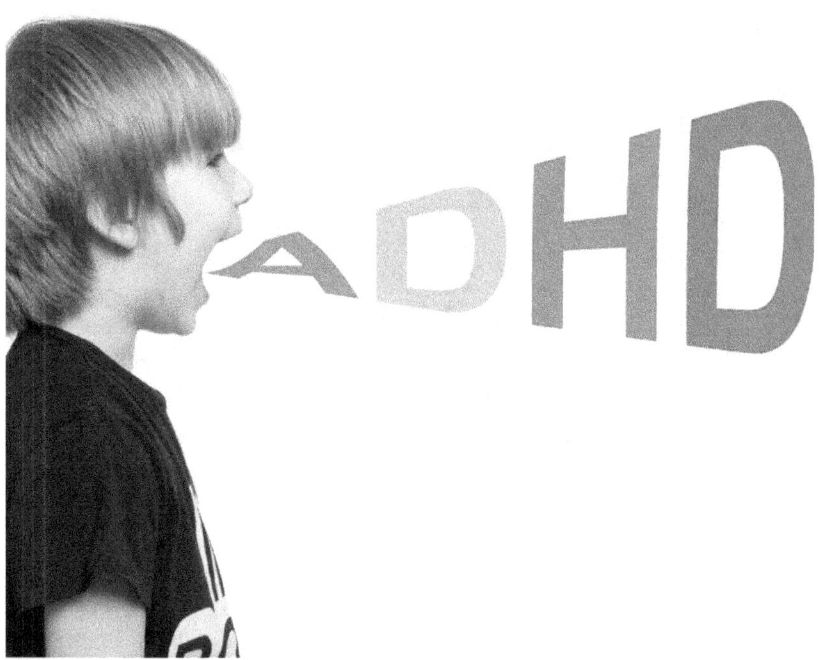

Attention Deficit Hyperactivity Disorder (ADHD) is a neurodevelopmental disorder characterized by a combination of inattentiveness, hyperactivity, and impulsivity. It is commonly diagnosed in childhood, but can persist into adulthood. ADHD is the most commonly diagnosed behavioral disorder in children and adolescents, and affects approximately 9.4 percent of children between the ages of 2 and 17 years old.

ADHD is caused by a combination of genetic and environmental factors. It is believed that a combination of genetic and environmental factors are responsible for the disorder, with the exact cause still unknown. Studies have shown that genetics is likely to play a role, as studies have found that individuals with ADHD have an increased risk of having a first-degree relative diagnosed with the disorder. Environmental factors, such as a lack of structure and parental guidance, as well as exposure to toxins, have also been found to be associated with the development of ADHD.

The primary symptoms of ADHD include inattention, impulsivity, and hyperactivity. Individuals with ADHD may have difficulty sustaining attention in tasks or activities, be easily distracted, and have difficulty organizing tasks or activities. They may also have difficulty controlling impulses, be overly talkative, and have difficulty sitting still for long periods of time.

Treatment for ADHD typically involves a combination of medication and behavioral strategies. Medication is often used to help control some of the symptoms of ADHD, such as impulsivity and hyperactivity. Behavioral strategies typically involve helping the individual to develop better organizational and time management skills, as well as providing an environment with structure and clear expectations.

While ADHD is a serious disorder, it is important to remember that it is treatable and individuals with ADHD can lead happy, productive lives. With the right treatment, individuals with ADHD can learn to manage their symptoms and live successful, fulfilling lives.

In conclusion, Attention Deficit Hyperactivity Disorder (ADHD) is a neurodevelopmental disorder characterized by a combination of inattentiveness, hyperactivity, and impulsivity. It is caused by a combination of genetic and environmental factors and is most commonly diagnosed in childhood. Treatment typically involves a combination of medication and behavioral strategies, and individuals with ADHD can lead successful, fulfilling lives with the right treatment and support.

Type of ADHD

ADHD is typically divided into three subtypes: predominantly inattentive, predominantly hyperactive-impulsive, and combined type.

The predominantly inattentive type is characterized by difficulty sustaining attention in tasks and activities, difficulty organizing tasks or activities, and difficulty following instructions.

The predominantly hyperactive-impulsive type is characterized by excessive talking, difficulty sitting still for long periods of time, and difficulty controlling impulsive behavior.

The combined type is characterized by symptoms of both the inattentive type and the hyperactive-impulsive type.

It is important to note that individuals may not fit neatly into one of these three subtypes and may exhibit symptoms from both types. Additionally, symptoms may vary over time and in different settings.

In conclusion, Attention Deficit Hyperactivity Disorder (ADHD) is a neurodevelopmental disorder characterized by a combination of inattentiveness, hyperactivity, and impulsivity. ADHD is typically divided into three subtypes: predominantly inattentive, predominantly hyperactive-impulsive, and combined type. It is caused by a combination of genetic and environmental factors and is most commonly diagnosed in childhood. Treatment typically involves a combination of medication and behavioral strategies, and individuals with ADHD can lead successful, fulfilling lives with the right treatment and support.

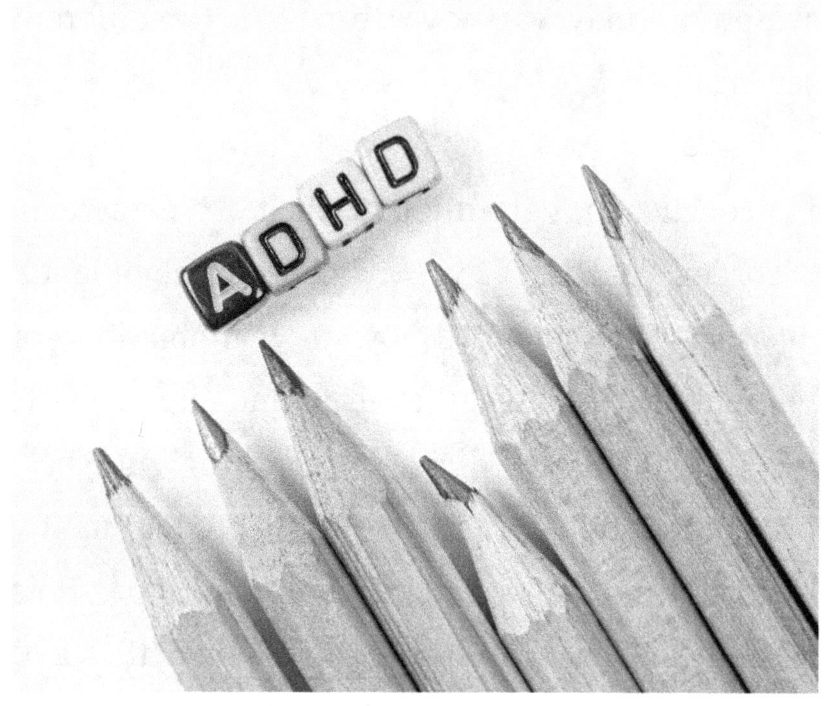

Chapter 2

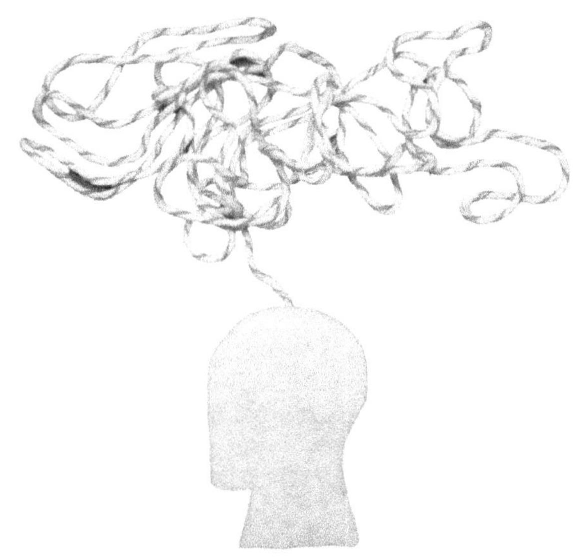

Attention Deficit Hyperactivity Disorder (ADHD) is a disorder that affects children and adults and is characterized by difficulty in paying attention, hyperactivity, and impulsivity. It is one of the most common mental health disorders in the United States and affects around 6.1 million children between the ages of 2 and 17.

ADHD is caused by a combination of genetic and environmental factors. The exact cause is not known, but it is believed to be related to a combination of factors including genetics, environmental factors, and brain chemistry.

ADHD affects the brain in a variety of ways. One of the main changes that occurs is in the prefrontal cortex, which is the area of the brain responsible for executive functioning. This area of the brain is responsible for planning, organization, decision making, and impulse control. In people with ADHD, this area of the brain does not function as well as it should, leading to the symptoms associated with the disorder.

ADHD can also affect the hippocampus, which is the area of the brain that is responsible for memory and learning. People with ADHD have difficulty focusing on tasks, paying attention, and remembering information. Additionally, they may have difficulty controlling their emotions, leading to emotional outbursts and difficulty regulating their behavior.

ADHD can also affect the dopamine system in the brain. Dopamine is a neurotransmitter that is responsible for motivation, reward, and pleasure. People with ADHD tend to have lower levels of dopamine, which can make it difficult to stay focused and motivated.

Finally, ADHD can also affect the basal ganglia, which is the area of the brain responsible for movement. People with ADHD often have difficulty controlling their movement, leading to hyperactivity and impulsivity.

Overall, ADHD can have a significant impact on the brain, leading to difficulty with executive functioning, memory, emotion regulation, and movement. Treatment for ADHD typically includes medication, behavioral therapy, and lifestyle changes to help manage symptoms.

If you or your child is showing signs of ADHD, it is important to talk to your doctor to discuss your options. With the right treatment and support, it is possible to reduce the impact of ADHD on your life.

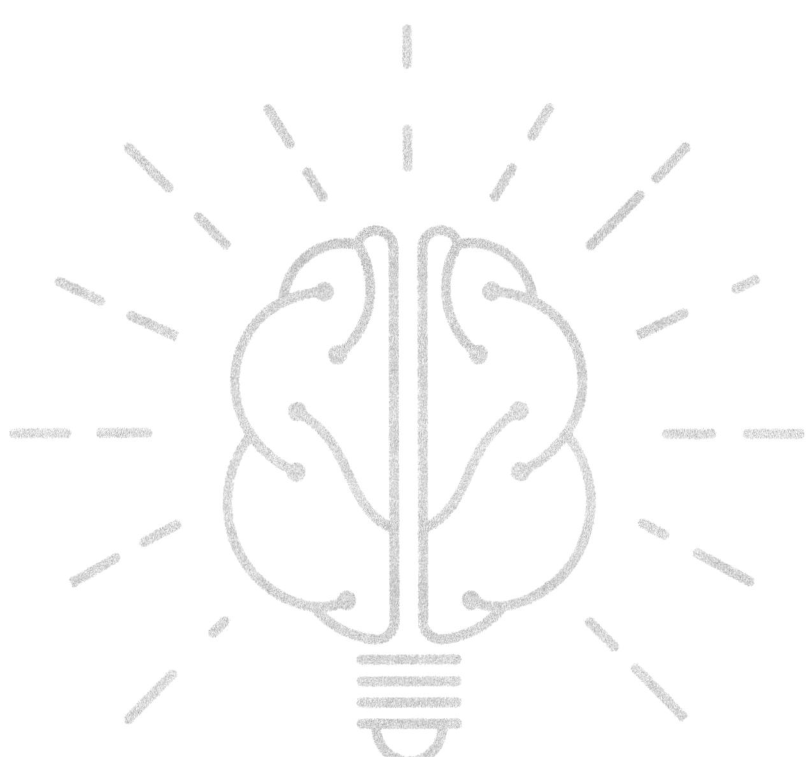

Chapter 3

Creating an ADHD-Friendly Home Environment

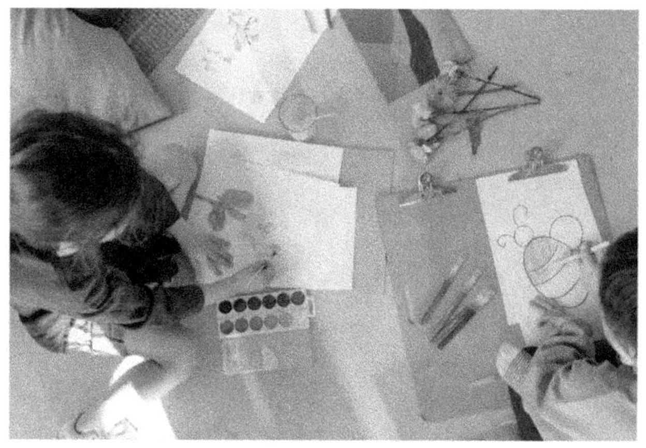

1. Prioritize Organization: A cluttered and disorganized living space can be overwhelming and stressful for children with ADHD, so make sure to create an organized and well-structured home environment. This can include labeling shelves and drawers, setting up a designated homework area, and creating a system for organizing toys and belongings.

2. Establish Routines: Establishing routines and expectations can help children with ADHD stay on task and provide structure. Try to set up a consistent daily schedule with dedicated time for homework, playtime, meals, chores, and bedtime.

3. Minimize Distractions: Minimize distractions in your home by reducing noise, turning off the TV, and removing toys and games that can be too stimulating for children with ADHD.

4. Provide Positive Reinforcement: Positive reinforcement is important for children with ADHD, so reward good behavior and provide praise for tasks that are completed.

5. Create an Outdoor Area: Creating an outdoor area for your child to play in can be a great way to

help them stay active and burn off extra energy. If possible, try to create a space that is fun and engaging, such as a backyard play area with a swing set, trampoline, or sandbox

6. Involve Your Child: Involve your child in the process of creating an ADHD-friendly home environment. Ask them for input on what activities they would like to do and what areas of the house they would like to organize. This can help your child feel more in control of their environment and give them a sense of ownership.

7. Get Professional Help: If your child's ADHD symptoms are severe and interfering with their daily life, seek the help of a mental health professional. They can provide additional strategies and resources to help your child manage their ADHD symptoms.

8. Be Patient: Creating an ADHD-friendly home environment can take some time, so be patient and take it one step at a time. With consistency and dedication, you can help create an environment that is conducive to your child's success.

Creating an ADHD-friendly home environment for your child is essential for helping them manage their symptoms and thrive. With some planning and guidance, you can create an organized, structured, and distraction-free home environment that is conducive to your child's success.

9. Set Boundaries: Setting consistent boundaries and expectations can help children with ADHD learn self-control and build self-esteem. Make sure

to clearly communicate expectations and provide consequences when boundaries are not followed.

10. Encourage Physical Activity: Regular physical activity can help children with ADHD manage their symptoms and stay focused. Encourage your child to get active by taking walks, playing sports, or participating in other activities.

11. Take Breaks: Taking regular breaks throughout the day can help children with ADHD stay focused and manage their symptoms. Encourage your child to take breaks throughout the day to give their brain a rest and help them recharge.

12. Connect with Other Families: Connecting with other families with children with ADHD can be a great way to get support and find resources. You can also use this opportunity to exchange tips and

advice, and learn more about how to create an ADHD-friendly home environment.

13. Get Enough Sleep: A lack of sleep can make ADHD symptoms worse, so make sure your child is getting enough rest. Establish a consistent bedtime routine and help create a calming environment for your child to relax and get the sleep they need.

14. Avoid Overstimulation: Overstimulation can make it harder for children with ADHD to focus, so try to create a calm and peaceful environment. Consider reducing screen time, turning off the TV, and limiting other activities that can be too stimulating.

15. Manage Stress: Stress can make it harder for children with ADHD to manage their symptoms, so find ways to help your child manage their stress.

This can include activities such as yoga, deep breathing, and mindfulness.

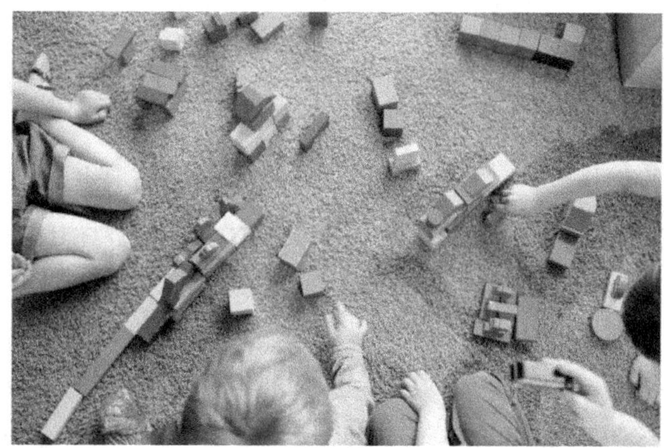

Chapter 4

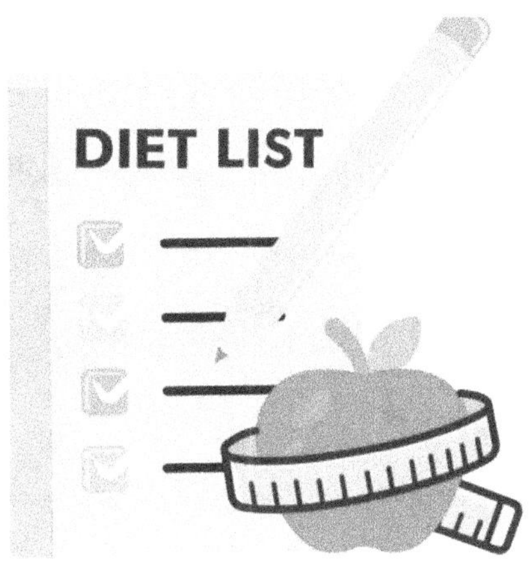

Diet is an important part of managing ADHD symptoms in children. Eating a balanced diet with plenty of fruits, vegetables, whole grains, lean proteins and healthy fats can help improve focus, reduce hyperactivity and improve overall behavior. Eating regular meals and snacks throughout the day can also help balance blood sugar levels, which can help reduce ADHD symptoms. Avoiding sugary, processed foods, artificial additives, and food dyes can also help prevent the worsening of symptoms. Additionally, omega-3 fatty acids, found in fish and certain plant sources, have been shown to reduce symptoms in some children. Finally, staying hydrated by drinking plenty of water throughout the day can help improve energy levels and concentration.

Meal plans

Day 1

Breakfast: Whole grain toast with peanut butter and banana slices

Snack: Carrot sticks and hummus

Lunch: Turkey wrap with lettuce, tomato, and avocado

Snack: Greek yogurt with blueberries

Dinner: Baked salmon with roasted asparagus and quinoa

Day 2

Breakfast: Overnight oats with chia seeds, almond milk, and berries

Snack: Apple slices with almond butter

Lunch: Quinoa salad with grilled chicken, cucumber, and tomatoes

Snack: Edamame

Dinner: Baked chicken with roasted sweet potatoes and broccoli

Day 3

Breakfast: Avocado toast with poached eggs and spinach

Snack: Celery sticks with nut butter

Lunch: Tuna salad wrap with lettuce, tomato, and cucumber

Snack: Air-popped popcorn

Dinner: Turkey burgers with roasted zucchini and sweet potato fries

Breakfast: Smoothie bowl with banana, almond milk, and chia seeds

Snack: Hard-boiled egg

Lunch: Grilled turkey and cheese sandwich with lettuce and tomato

Snack: Whole grain crackers with hummus

Dinner: Baked salmon with roasted Brussels sprouts and brown rice

Breakfast: Oatmeal with banana slices and walnuts

Snack: Greek yogurt with berries

Lunch: Quinoa salad with grilled chicken, cucumber, and tomatoes

Snack: Apple slices with nut butter

Dinner: Baked chicken with roasted asparagus and sweet potatoes

Day 6

Breakfast: Whole grain toast with peanut butter and banana slices

Snack: Carrot sticks and hummus

Lunch: Turkey wrap with lettuce, tomato, and avocado

Snack: Edamame

Dinner: Baked salmon with roasted Brussels sprouts and quinoa

Day 7

Breakfast: Overnight oats with chia seeds, almond milk, and berries

Snack: Greek yogurt with blueberries

Lunch: Quinoa salad with grilled chicken, cucumber, and tomatoes

Snack: Air-popped popcorn

Dinner: Turkey burgers with roasted zucchini and sweet potato fries

Breakfast: Avocado toast with poached eggs and spinach

Snack: Celery sticks with nut butter

Lunch: Tuna salad wrap with lettuce, tomato, and cucumber

Snack: Whole grain crackers with hummus

Dinner: Baked salmon with roasted asparagus and brown rice

Day 9

Breakfast: Smoothie bowl with banana, almond milk, and chia seeds

Snack: Hard-boiled egg

Lunch: Grilled turkey and cheese sandwich with lettuce and tomato

Snack: Apple slices with nut butter

Dinner: Baked chicken with roasted Brussels sprouts and sweet potatoes

Day 10

Breakfast: Oatmeal with banana slices and walnuts

Snack: Greek yogurt with berries

Lunch: Quinoa salad with grilled chicken, cucumber, and tomatoes

Snack: Carrot sticks and hummus

Dinner: Baked salmon with roasted asparagus and quinoa in and diet for children

Breakfast: Whole wheat pancakes with fresh fruit

Snack: Trail mix

Lunch: Lentil soup with whole grain bread

Snack: Celery with nut butter

Dinner: Baked tofu with roasted vegetables and quinoa

Breakfast: Omelette with spinach and tomatoes

Snack: Smoothie with almond milk and banana

Lunch: Grilled chicken sandwich with avocado and lettuce

Snack: Edamame

Dinner: Baked cod with roasted potatoes and broccoli

Day 13

Breakfast: Oatmeal with walnuts and banana slices

Snack: Greek yogurt with blueberries

Lunch: Quinoa salad with grilled chicken, cucumber, and tomatoes

Snack: Whole grain crackers with hummus

Dinner: Baked turkey with roasted asparagus and sweet potatoes

Day 14

Breakfast: Whole grain toast with peanut butter and banana slices

Snack: Carrot sticks and hummus

Lunch: Turkey wrap with lettuce, tomato, and avocado

Snack: Apple slices with nut butter

Dinner: Baked salmon with roasted Brussels sprouts and quinoa

Breakfast: Smoothie bowl with banana, almond milk, and chia seeds

Snack: Hard-boiled egg

Lunch: Grilled turkey and cheese sandwich with lettuce and tomato

Snack: Air-popped popcorn

Dinner: Baked chicken with roasted zucchini and sweet potato fries

Breakfast: Avocado toast with poached eggs and spinach

Snack: Celery sticks with nut butter

Lunch: Tuna salad wrap with lettuce, tomato, and cucumber

Snack: Greek yogurt with berries

Dinner: Baked salmon with roasted asparagus and brown rice

Day 17

Breakfast: Overnight oats with chia seeds, almond milk, and berries

Snack: Apple slices with almond butter

Lunch: Quinoa salad with grilled chicken, cucumber, and tomatoes

Snack: Edamame

Dinner: Baked chicken with roasted sweet potatoes and broccoli

Breakfast: Oatmeal with banana slices and walnuts

Snack: Whole grain crackers with hummus

Lunch: Turkey wrap with lettuce, tomato, and avocado

Snack: Carrot sticks with hummus

Dinner: Baked salmon with roasted Brussels sprouts and quinoa

Breakfast: Smoothie bowl with banana, almond milk, and chia seeds

Snack: Hard-boiled egg

Lunch: Grilled turkey and cheese sandwich with lettuce and tomato

Snack: Apple slices with nut butter

Dinner: Baked chicken with roasted asparagus and sweet potatoes

Breakfast: Avocado toast with poached eggs and spinach

Snack: Celery sticks with nut butter

Lunch: Tuna salad wrap with lettuce, tomato, and cucumber

Snack: Greek yogurt with blueberries

Dinner: Baked salmon with roasted zucchini and brown rice

Day 21

Breakfast: Oatmeal with banana slices and walnuts

Snack: Trail mix

Lunch: Quinoa salad with grilled chicken, cucumber, and tomatoes

Snack: Air-popped popcorn

Dinner: Turkey burgers with roasted asparagus and sweet potato fries

Day 22

Breakfast: Whole wheat pancakes with fresh fruit

Snack: Hard-boiled egg

Lunch: Lentil soup with whole grain bread

Snack: Whole grain crackers with hummus

Dinner: Baked tofu with roasted vegetables and quinoa

Day 23

Breakfast: Omelette with spinach and tomatoes

Snack: Smoothie with almond milk and banana

Lunch: Grilled chicken sandwich with avocado and lettuce

Snack: Edamame

Dinner: Baked cod with roasted potatoes and broccoli

Day 24

Breakfast: Overnight oats with chia seeds, almond milk, and berries

Snack: Carrot sticks and hummus

Lunch: Turkey wrap with lettuce, tomato, and avocado

Snack: Apple slices with nut butter

Dinner: Baked salmon with roasted Brussels sprouts and quinoa

Day 25

Breakfast: Whole grain toast with peanut butter and banana slices

Snack: Greek yogurt with berries

Lunch: Quinoa salad with grilled chicken, cucumber, and tomatoes

Snack: Celery with nut butter

Dinner: Baked chicken with roasted asparagus and sweet potatoes

Breakfast: Smoothie bowl with banana, almond milk, and chia seeds

Snack: Hard-boiled egg

Lunch: Grilled turkey and cheese sandwich with lettuce and tomato

Snack: Air-popped popcorn

Dinner: Baked salmon with roasted zucchini and brown rice

Day 27

Breakfast: Oatmeal with walnuts and banana slices

Snack: Greek yogurt with blueberries

Lunch: Quinoa salad with grilled chicken, cucumber, and tomatoes

Snack: Whole grain crackers with hummus

Dinner: Baked turkey with roasted asparagus and sweet potatoes

Day 28

Breakfast: Avocado toast with poached eggs and spinach

Snack: Carrot sticks and hummus

Lunch: Tuna salad wrap with lettuce, tomato, and cucumber

Snack: Apple slices with nut butter

Dinner: Baked salmon with roasted Brussels sprouts and quinoa

Day 29

Breakfast: Whole wheat pancakes with fresh fruit

Snack: Trail mix

Lunch: Lentil soup with whole grain bread

Snack: Edamame

Dinner: Baked tofu with roasted vegetables and quinoa

Day 30

Breakfast: Omelette with spinach and tomatoes

Snack: Smoothie with almond milk and banana

Lunch: Grilled chicken sandwich with avocado and lettuce

Snack: Celery with nut butter

Dinner: Baked cod with roasted potatoes and broccoli

Chapter 5

Exercise and ADHD

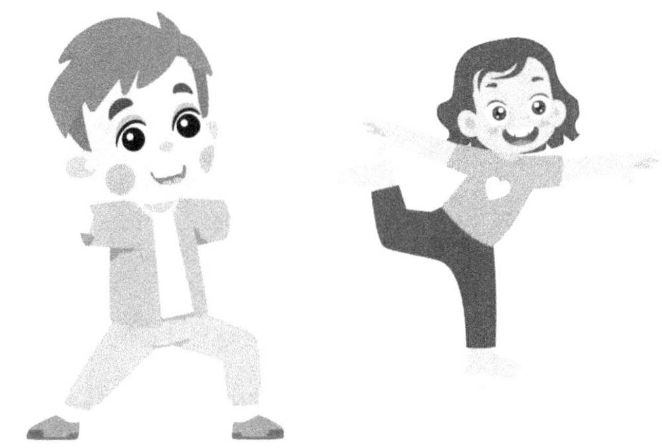

Exercise can be an important part of managing attention deficit hyperactivity disorder (ADHD) in children. Research has shown that physical activity can improve focus, reduce impulsivity, and boost self-esteem in children with ADHD. Exercise has also been found to help reduce the symptoms of hyperactivity, inattention, and impulsivity.

Regular physical activity can help children with ADHD maintain focus and concentration, manage their emotions, and improve their overall behavior. Exercise can also help reduce stress and anxiety, which often accompany ADHD. Additionally, physical activity can help improve sleep, which is often disrupted in children with ADHD.

In addition to the physical benefits of exercise, it can also provide children with ADHD an outlet to express themselves and gain confidence. Exercise can help children with ADHD learn to manage their emotions and increase their self-esteem. Participating in physical activities can also lead to improved social skills since it provides an opportunity to interact with other children and practice problem-solving.

To maximize the benefits of physical activity, children with ADHD should engage in activities that they enjoy and find motivating. This could include sports, martial arts, swimming, or riding a bike. It is also important to ensure that children have breaks when needed and avoid overdoing it. Regular physical activity is key for children with ADHD, so parents should encourage their children to be active and monitor how much exercise they are getting.

Ultimately, exercise can be an important part of managing ADHD in children. By providing physical, mental, and emotional benefits, exercise can help children with ADHD improve their focus, reduce impulsivity, and boost their self-esteem.

Type of Exercise for ADHD children

The type of exercise that is best for children with ADHD depends on the individual child and their particular needs. Some activities that are beneficial for children with ADHD include running, swimming, biking, martial arts, and team sports.

Running is a great way to help children with ADHD manage their energy levels and focus. It can also help improve their overall physical fitness. Swimming is also a great activity for children with ADHD as it helps to improve coordination, focus, and concentration. Biking is another great activity for children with ADHD as it helps to increase physical endurance and improve balance.

Martial arts can be a great way for children with ADHD to learn self-discipline and focus. It can also help improve coordination and self-confidence. Team sports can help children with ADHD learn to interact with others and practice problem-solving. It also encourages physical activity and helps to improve physical fitness. Ultimately, the type of exercise that is best for children with ADHD depends on the individual child and their particular needs. It is important to find activities that the child enjoys and feels motivated to do in order to get the most out of it. By providing physical, mental, and emotional benefits, exercise can help children with ADHD improve their focus, reduce impulsivity, and boost their self-esteem.

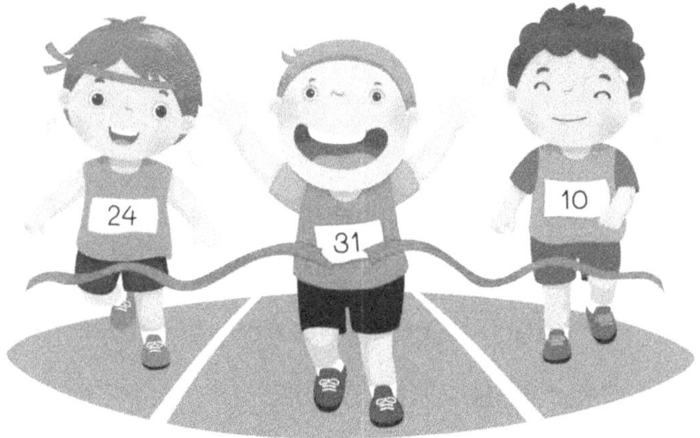

Chapter 6

Organizational Strategies for ADHD

1. Establish a routine: Having a consistent daily routine can help reduce the chance of forgetting assignments or having difficulty managing time.

2. Break tasks down into smaller components: Breaking tasks down into smaller, more manageable components can make them less overwhelming and help kids with ADHD focus and stay on track.

3. Use visual reminders: Posting visual reminders where they can be seen and easily referenced can be helpful for kids with ADHD.

4. Use short breaks: Short breaks can help kids with ADHD refocus and stay on task.

5. Provide rewards and incentives: Rewarding good behavior and providing incentives for completing tasks can help motivate kids with ADHD.

6. Allow for flexibility: Allowing for some flexibility in the structure of tasks can help kids with ADHD stay engaged and motivated.

7. Utilize technology: Technology, such as timers, apps, and organizers, can be helpful for kids with ADHD as it can help them stay organized and on track.

8. Offer structure: Offering structure and consistent expectations can help kids with ADHD stay focused and on task.

9. Use positive reinforcement: Positive reinforcement of desired behaviors can help kids with ADHD stay motivated and engaged.

10. Have a plan for times of stress: Having a plan for when things get overwhelming can help kids with ADHD stay focused and on task.

11. Provide accommodations: Providing accommodations, such as extra time or preferential seating, can help kids with ADHD succeed.

12. Seek help: Seeking out help from professionals can be beneficial for kids with ADHD.

13. Support involvement in activities: Supporting involvement in activities outside of school can help

kids with ADHD build self-esteem and stay motivated.

14. Encourage self-advocacy: Teaching kids with ADHD to advocate for themselves can help them become more confident and successful.

15. Model good behavior: Modeling good behavior and positive reinforcement can help kids with ADHD stay on task and motivated.

16. Use study strategies: Using study strategies, such as chunking and mnemonics, can help kids with ADHD stay organized and on task.

17. Encourage goal setting: Encouraging kids with ADHD to set goals for themselves can help them stay focused and motivated.

18. Foster relationships: Foster relationships with teachers, peers and other adults can help kids with ADHD stay engaged and motivated.

19. Practice self-care: Practicing self-care can help kids with ADHD stay focused and on task, as well as reduce stress and anxiety.

20. Connect with other parents: Connecting with other parents of kids with ADHD can help provide support and understanding.

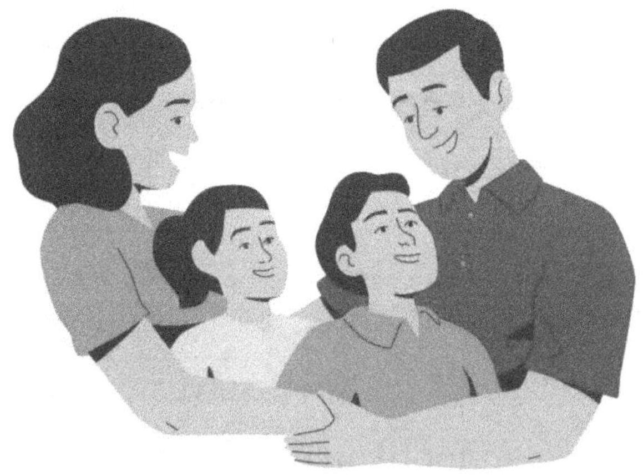

Chapter 7

Managing Time and Schedules

1. Break tasks into manageable chunks: Break down large tasks into smaller, more easily achievable pieces. This can help ADHD children stay focused and on task.

2. Use visual cues: ADHD children often benefit from visual cues to help them stay on track with their tasks. Use pictures, diagrams, or anything else that helps them keep their focus.

3. Set a routine: Establishing a regular routine can help ADHD children stay organized and on task. Make sure to leave time for breaks and fun activities.

4. Prioritize tasks: ADHD children may have difficulty prioritizing tasks. Help them prioritize by breaking down tasks into smaller pieces and deciding which ones need to be done first.

5. Use a timer: Setting a timer for tasks can help ADHD children stay focused. Give them a set amount of time to complete tasks, and then reward them for a job well done.

6. Set expectations: Make sure ADHD children understand expectations for completing tasks, and the consequences for not doing so. This can help them stay on track and motivated.

7. Get help: If needed, reach out to a professional who can help provide strategies to help an ADHD child manage their time and schedules.

8. Provide rewards: Provide rewards for completing tasks. This can help encourage ADHD children to stay on task and motivated.

9. Take breaks: Taking regular breaks can help ADHD children stay focused and energized. Make sure to provide them with activities that are stimulating yet calming.

10. Stay positive: Encouragement and positive reinforcement can go a long way in helping ADHD children manage their time and schedules.

Chapter 8

ADHD and Social Skills

1. Model positive social skills: Children learn best by watching adults model the behavior they want them to emulate. Show your child polite manners, demonstrate how to introduce themselves to others, and talk to them about appropriate social behavior.

2. Practice social skills in different settings: Role play common social interactions with your child, such as introducing themselves to others, taking turns in conversations, and making small talk. This helps your child become more comfortable in different social situations.

3. Encourage participation in group activities: Being part of a group, such as a sports team, can help children with ADHD develop better social skills. It provides an opportunity for them to practice interacting with others, following directions, and working as part of a team.

4. Talk about emotions: Help your child understand and recognize their emotions, as well as the emotions of others. Explain how different emotions can lead to different reactions in social situations.

5. Set appropriate boundaries: Establish expectations and rules for your child's social interactions. This will help them understand acceptable behavior and give them the tools they need to practice appropriate social skills.

6. Provide feedback: Let your child know when they are engaging in positive social behaviors, and give them feedback on how to improve when needed. Praise your child for their efforts and remind them that practice makes perfect.

7. Encourage positive relationships: Help your child foster relationships with other children and adults. Encourage them to talk about their interests, practice active listening skills, and engage in conversations.

8. Spend time with your child: Make an effort to spend quality time with your child. This will help them build confidence and trust, and will give you an opportunity to reinforce the social skills you've been teaching.

9. Seek professional help: If your child is having difficulty with social skills, consider seeking the help of a mental health professional. They can provide individualized interventions to help your child develop the skills they need to succeed in social settings.

10. Stay positive: Being a parent of a child with ADHD can be challenging, but staying positive is key. Modeling good social skills and maintaining a positive attitude will help your child learn and practice the necessary skills.

Chapter 9

Dealing with Bullying

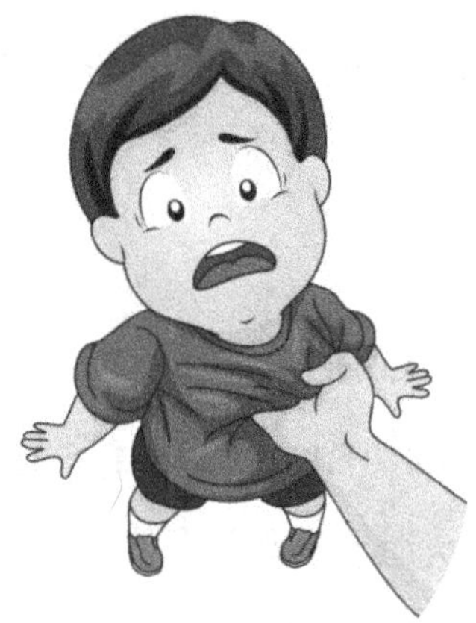

1. Talk to your child: Let your child know that it's okay to talk to you about difficult topics, like being bullied. Ask them how they feel and listen without judgment.

2.Set boundaries: Help your child understand that they don't have to accept the bullying and that they have the right to stand up for themselves.

3.Encourage positive coping: Teach your child positive coping strategies to deal with the bullying, such as deep breathing, talking to a trusted adult, or finding other activities to help them relax.

4.Teach your child social skills: If your child has difficulty making friends or understanding social norms, consider enrolling them in a social skills group.

5.Teach your child self-advocacy: Help your child learn to advocate for themselves in situations where they don't feel safe.

6.Get support: Reach out to other parents, teachers, and counselors for support and advice.

7.Get help from professionals: If the bullying persists, seek help from a mental health professional who specializes in ADHD.

8.Stay in contact with school: Stay in touch with the school and ensure that they are taking appropriate steps to address the bullying.

9.Encourage participation in activities: Encourage your child to participate in activities that they enjoy and that are outside of school. This will help them develop positive connections with peers.

10.Be a role model: Show your child that you are willing to stand up for yourself and others in the face of bullying. This will help them learn to do the same.

Chapter 10

Living with ADHD

Living with ADHD as a parent of a child with the disorder can be very difficult. Parents may feel overwhelmed, frustrated, and exhausted by the constant demands of managing the condition. ADHD can affect a child's ability to pay attention and focus, to stay on task, to regulate their emotions, and to interact with peers appropriately. Parents may need to help their child set daily goals, use positive reinforcement to encourage positive behaviors, and provide structure and routine. It is also important for parents to take care of themselves and seek out support from professionals, family, and friends.

It is also important for parents to be aware of potential side effects of medication, monitor their child's progress, and be mindful of their child's feelings and needs. Parents should be aware that ADHD is a lifelong disorder and may require ongoing treatment and support. Additionally, parents should remember that their child is not defined by their diagnosis and can still achieve their dreams.

Finally, it is important for parents to remember that they are not alone. There are many resources available to families living with ADHD and many organizations that offer support and guidance.

Conclusion

Taking Charge of Your ADHD

1. Set Boundaries: Establish clear boundaries for your child and make sure they understand what is expected of them. Be consistent with your expectations and enforce the rules.

2. Provide Structure: Structure is important for children to learn how to manage their time and responsibilities. Having a daily routine, such as regular mealtimes, bedtimes, and activities, will help your child to feel secure and organized.

3. Encourage Responsibility: Teaching your child responsibility is key to helping them become independent and self-sufficient. Encourage them

to take on tasks and responsibilities, such as helping with chores, and offer rewards when they complete them.

4. Monitor Screen Time: Too much screen time can have a negative effect on your child's development. Set limits on their electronic use and provide alternatives for them to engage in more productive activities.

5. Listen and Respond: Take the time to listen to your child and respond to their needs and feelings. Respect their thoughts and feelings and be sure to give them a chance to voice their opinions.

6. Foster Healthy Habits: Help your child develop healthy habits, such as exercise, eating healthy foods, and getting enough rest. Be a good role model and lead by example.

7. Celebrate Achievements: Praise your child when they accomplish something, big or small. Celebrate their successes and let them know that you're proud of them.

8. Be Supportive: Be understanding and supportive of your child. Encourage them to take on new challenges and provide them with the resources they need to succeed.

9. Show Love and Affection: Show your child that you love and care for them by spending quality time together and showing affection. Let them know that you're there for them and that you will always be their biggest supporter.

10. Seek Help: If you're having difficulty managing your child, don't be afraid to seek help from professionals such as counselors or therapists.